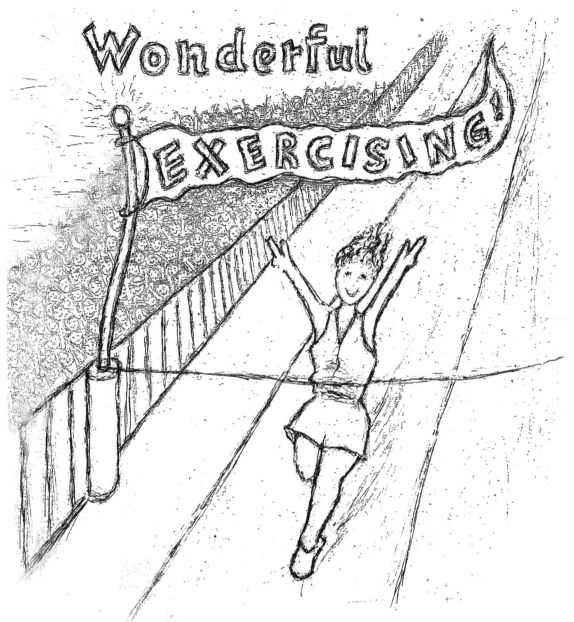

Wonderful EXERCISING!

A Fitness-Mini-Series with Illustrations!

TANYA LIESL HERRERE

authorHOUSE

AuthorHouse™
1663 Liberty Drive
Bloomington, IN 47403
www.authorhouse.com
Phone: 1 (800) 839-8640

Published by AuthorHouse 11/23/2019

ISBN: 978-1-7283-3293-2 (sc)
ISBN: 978-1-7283-3292-5 (e)

Print information available on the last page.

Any people depicted in stock imagery provided by Getty Images are models, and such images are being used for illustrative purposes only. Certain stock imagery © Getty Images.

Scripture quotations marked KJV are from the Holy Bible, King James Version (Authorized Version). First published in 1611. Quoted from the KJV Classic Reference Bible, Copyright © 1983 by The Zondervan Corporation.

This book is printed on acid-free paper.

Because of the dynamic nature of the Internet, any web addresses or links contained in this book may have changed since publication and may no longer be valid. The views expressed in this work are solely those of the author and do not necessarily reflect the views of the publisher, and the publisher hereby disclaims any responsibility for them.

Introduction

Show me thy ways, O LORD: teach me thy path.
Psalm: 25, 4

Wonderful Exercising could well be called a 'Fitness-Program-With-Hope; for it could bring new hope to many of us who always wanted something more enjoyable and lasting in the way of exercising. To make a stab into a new direction, we are hereby invited to take a look at this unique working model. But let's remember, it's not so much in the 'looking' but much more in the 'doing and practicing' of the actual work-out-session, in that we can experience its true value and success!

Basically, the program is rather a combination of some physical-mental- and spiritual-forces working together, including at times-a bit of deep-breathing.

The bulk of the session is made up of twelve continuous episodes in sequence; there by creating a playful 'Mini-Series', in which any one of us can become the 'Star of the Show'!

All of the episodes come with a 'back-up-script'. The script can be interesting in providing information about: structure, benefits, and even a bit about history of various exercises involved.

The actual work-out-session can be accomplished in more or less one-hour. In this relatively short time, we can have a good physical-work-out, as well have some fun-experiences along the way; And all of this, by just using our own creative-mental and spiritual resources.

Last and most importantly: Wonderful Exercising would like to make it known that every precious Psalm-Verse that is featured in the program is exactly the same as it is written in the King James Version.

With such good company at our side can there be any doubt that we will have a most wonderful exercising-experience in store for us?

O LORD my God, I will give thanks unto thee forever.
Psalm: 30, 12

A Place to Exercise!

The Program can give us two great options!

<u>First-Option:</u> We can actually do our first six Episodes right on our very own 'Bed' with the cover put-aside! Our next six finishing-Episodes we can do right next to our 'Bed' with a chair and our work-book nearby! This maybe especially "Good News" for our seniors, who rather like to stay on top of things! O Happy Day!

<u>Another Option:</u> We may just find a good spot around the house where we can spread out our 'Exercising pad' and have a bit of room to move: A chair nearby and a window-open can be helpful again to have a good 'Exercising-Place' to enjoy!

<u>Things to Remember:</u> Let's keep counting (audibly or manually)! Counting can be helpful to maintain the structure and discipline for any good program to be successful! Remembering also the 'positive-mental-imagery-the 'Breathing'-and the 'Speaking' of the lovely 'Psalm-verses' while exercising! All of which can make our exercising time so much more enjoyable and successful!

Wonderful-Exercising!
Beginning of the Workout!

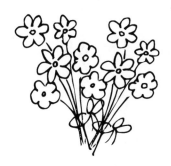

A Mini-Series in 12 Episodes
Time-Span of the Entire session Approx. One Hour

SCRIPT for EPISODE: 1

Presenting: <u>'Swing-Up and Breathe!</u>

We will be starting our First EPISODE with seven-'Warm-Up-Swings', which will bring us directly into a certain 'Back-Rest-Position'! (See Illustr.)

While in that 'position' it is important to do a bit of 'Breathing'-deeply and slowly, (about 4 to 5 times). We may also speak some of our favoured-Psalm-verses to go along with the 'Exercise' and the 'breathing'!

All of this could bring about a few good Extra-Benefits as for instance:

1) Increase of circulation in the 'Back-Area'!
2) A stronger flow of 'oxygen' toward the 'Chest and Brain-Area!
3) Elevation of positive-emotional-effects which can be helpful for fighting light depressions!

A few warm-up swings can bring us directly into Episode 2

EPISODE: 1 - Action!

"Blessed be the LORD, who dayly kindeth us with benefits."
Psalm: 68-19.

'Swing-Up' and 'Breathe'!
Psalm: 27-1-4

THE LORD is my light and my salvation; whom shall I fear? the LORD is the strength of my life; of whom shall I be afraid?

When the wicked, even mine enemies and my foes came upon me to eat up my flesh, they stumbled and fell.

Though an host should encamp against me, my heart shall not fear: though war should rise against me, in this will I be confident.

One thing have I desired of the LORD, that I will seek after, that I may dwell in the house of the LORD all the days of my life, to behold the beauty of the LORD, and to inquire in his temple.

We may have our own favorite
Psalm-verse or meditation
to go along with the exercise!
The choice is ours!

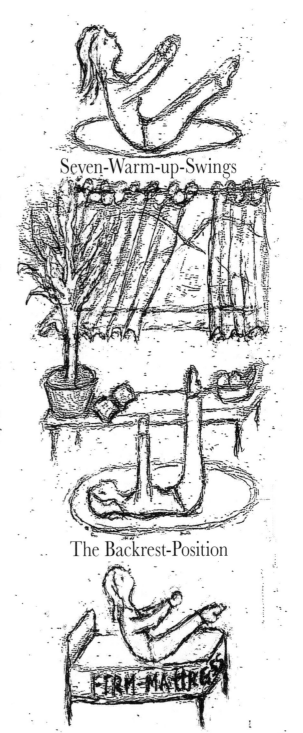

Seven-Warm-up-Swings

The Backrest-Position

SCRIPT FOR EPISODE: 2

Presenting: <u>'A Combination of Three'</u>!

Three Basic-Exercise-Positions are working from one-into the other-there-by creating a powerful 'Work-Out-Combination'!

1) <u>The 'Pouch'</u>: a rather interesting exercise which can work simultaneously on 'back-muscles'-'tummy-muscles'-all the way up to the neck and chin-area! The Pouch could be helpful-in time-to prevent double-chin and sagging effects.

2) <u>The 'Tummy-Squeeze'</u>: It is always working hard to keep the mid-section strong and flat.

3) <u>'The Lower-Back-Lift</u>: It is most effective with 'Breathing'! It can greatly strengthen the lower-back-muscles-and thereby prevent back pain, which can be caused by week muscles.

EPISODE 2 - Action!

"Thou hast commanded us to keep thy precepts diligently."
Psalm 119, 4

<u>A Combination of Three:</u>

<u>The Pouch:</u> Cuddle up - breathe in deeply: Hold breath pouching cheeks while lifting head and shoulders - while up turn head to the right and blow a bit of air from the right corner of the mouth turn head to the left and do the same in that direction lay back down and breathe out completely.
(Repeat 7 times!)

<u>The Tummy-squeeze:</u> Lay back with knees pushed up and feet placed on flat surface - with arms extended towards the knees - push upper-torso quickly back and forth!
(From 7 to 21 squeezes can have great results.)

<u>The Lower-back-lift:</u> Lay back with knees pushed-up and feet placed flat on surface; breathe in deeply while lifting your lower - back upwardly, held position and breath while counting to seven gently lower back down again while breathing out completely!
(Repeat procedure 7 times!)

Seven warm-up-swings will swing us directly into the next feature

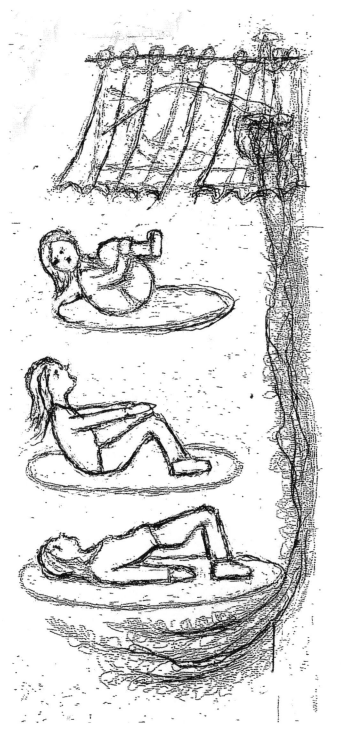

SCRIPT FOR EPISODE: 3

Presenting: <u>'Sit 'n' Speak'!</u>

While sitting-up for Episode 3, we will be doing three exercising-positions which are rather simple, however each one will have something important to say:

When we are speaking and repeating some of the words from Psalm: 139, 14: We may thereby remember again the awesome care and wonder invested in our very being!

All of this could make us more aware and remind us, to be more careful about ourselves! We might even remember some others who may need a bit of extra-T.L.C.!

A few warm-up-swings can bring us directly into Episode: 4

EPISODE 3 - Action!

"Thy word is a lamp unto my feet, and a light unto my path"
Psalm 119, 35

"I will praise thee; for I am fearfully and wonderfully made!" Reaching from our head, all the way to our feet, while speaking part of Psalm: 139, 14 - (Repeat: 5 to 7-times)

Turning from side to side with a little hug, while speaking something positive: "I'll be good to myself" or "I'll be joyful today"! (Repeat 5-7 times)

Open our arms wide while speaking: "I'll be careful for others"- or-"I'll be good to others"! (Repeat: 5-7 times)

A Little Scalp-Massage will end our Episode happily!

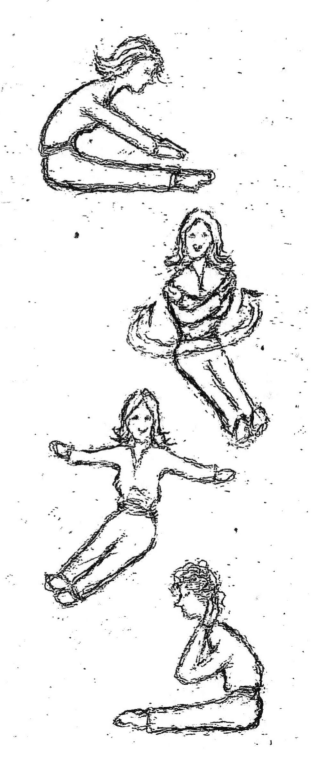

SCRIPT FOR EPISODE: 4

Presenting: <u>'Bicycling in the Country'</u>!

Leaning back now, we may be ready for a little 'Bicycle-Ride'! It may be important now to do a bit of 'Positive-Imaging'! As for instance: 'Perhaps we can remember a special-fun-time in the past. 'Riding along 'Happy-go-Lucky' with friends along a Beautiful Country Road! It's spring-time! Trees and flowers are blooming – the sky is blue! Soon we may discover a green meadow where we can stretch-out now and do a bit of 'good breathing' while speaking some lovely verses from Psalm: 23! All of which can create for us again another enjoyable Exercising-Experience!

A few warm-up-swings may swing us into our first Re-Run!

EPISODE: 4 - Action!

"Thy drop upon the pasture of the wilderness; and the little hills rejoice on every side." Psalm: 65:12,

Bicycling in the Country

We'll be pedaling on our back 100 cycles; counting fast (5x20) using five fingers one for each count of twenty; while reflecting on a bicycling-outing into the country-side.

Psalm: 23

The LORD is my shepherd; I shall not want.

He maketh me to lie down in green pastures: he leadeth me beside the still waters.

He restoreth my soul: He leadeth me in the path of righteousness for his name's sake.

Yea, though I walk through the valley of the shadow of death, I will fear no evil: for thou art with me; thy rod and thy staff they comfort me.

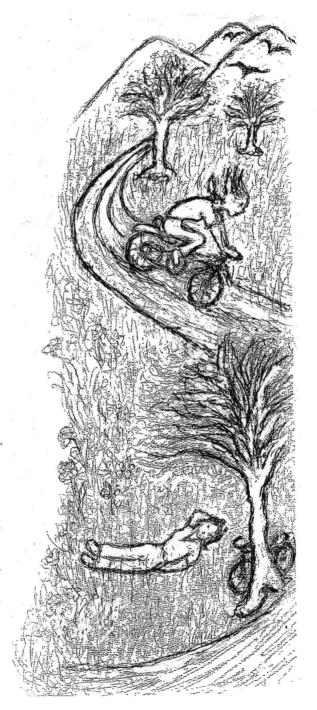

Thou preparest a table before me in the presence or mine enemies. Thou anointest my head with oil; my cup runneth over.

Surely goodness and mercy shall follow me all the days of my life: and I will dwell in the house of the LORD for ever.

"Breathe deeply while speaking some of the lovely Psalm.

RE-RUN of EPISODE 2

Presenting: <u>A Combination of Three!</u>

Three basic 'Exercise-Positions' are working from one into the other, thereby creating a powerful-Work-out-Combination!

1) <u>The Pouch</u> is rather interesting, because it can work simultaneous on some tummy muscles and back-muscles-all the way up to the neck-and-chin-area. It can be helpful to prevent-in time –'Double-chin and 'Sagging'-effects!
2) <u>The Tummy-Squeeze</u> is always working hard to keep the mid-section strong and flat.
3) <u>The Lower-Back-Lift</u> is just so effective with 'breathing'! It can greatly strengthen the 'Lower-Back-Muscles, and thereby prevent back pain which can be caused by week muscles.

Re-Run-I

"Thou hast commanded as to keep thy precepts diligently"
Psalm 119, 4

<u>A Combination of Three:</u>

<u>The Pouch</u> Cuddle up - breathe in deeply breath pouching cheeks while lifting head and shoulders - while up turn head to the right and blow, a bit of air from the right corner of the mouth turn head to the left and do the same in that direction: lay back down and breathe out completely.
(Repeat 7 times!)

<u>The Tummy-squeeze:</u> Lay back with knees pushed and feet placed on flat surface with arms extended towards the knees - push upper torso quickly back and forth!
(From 7 to 21 squeezes can have great results.)

<u>The Lower-back-lift:</u> Lay back with knees pushed-up and feet placed flat on surface: breathe in deeply while lifting your lower back upwardly hold position and breath while counting to seven gently lower back down again while breathing out completely!
(Repeat procedure 7 times!)

Seven warm-up-swings will swing us directly into the next feature)

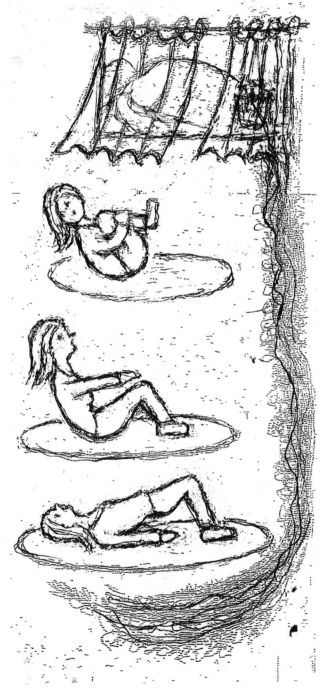

13

SCRIPT FOR EPISODE: 5

Presenting: <u>A Trip to the Sea-Shore!</u>

After our Re-Run, it will be fun to have another little Bicycle-Trip to the Beach! Pedaling our 100-cycles, we might already see that great blue ocean in the distance, shimmering, and inviting us, to come down into that soft-warm sand and do our exercises. While watching the waves, the children, and all the fun things going on around the beautiful 'sea-shore': "And see the wondres evening-sky-the glowing sun beyond the cliffs from where the seagulls come a sweeping down into the dark and shiny sea-to fetch the evening-meal, and back they fly, to feed their waiting young!"

A few warm-up-swings will bring us into our next Episode: 6

EPISODE: 5 - Action!

He giveth to the beast his food and to the
young ravens which cry: Ps: 147

A Trip to the Sea-Shore!

We pedal 100 fast cycles
counting:
Threw-hands-fall: 20 for each
fingers while anticipating the
beautiful sea-shore

Work-out in the Sand!

The Side-Kicks!
While stretched out on
our side, kicking up one leg—
counting audibly-between 7 to
21 times, while reflecting upon
a happy beach-day: "Watching
the waves come rolling in.
Turned around now, we can
exercise the other leg. While
watching the children play while
building their beautiful sand-castles!

The Cross-Kicks!
On our back and propped up
on our elbows:
On swinging one leg over the
other, counting between 7 and
21 cross-kicks for each leg; while
looking up turning out head
leisurely following the sea-birds
in their flight!

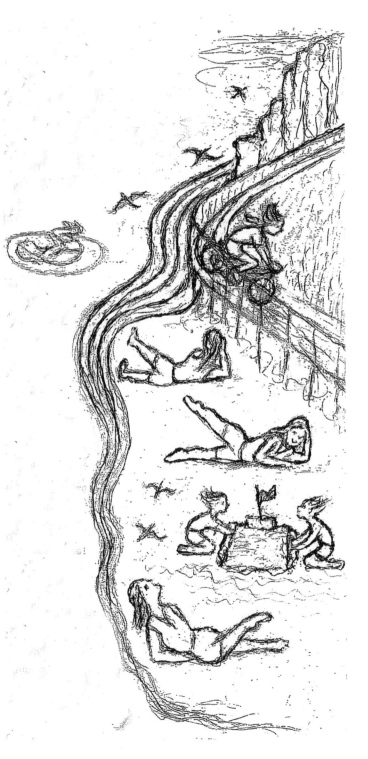

15

SCRIPT: FOR EPISODE: 6

Presenting: <u>'Swing High' - 'Swing Low'</u>!

Episode: 6 is providing for us two options!

For One: <u>"Swing-High"</u> could have a few good benefits in store for us, as for instance:

1) Better circulation for the - 'Upper-chest-and-neck-area'!
2) Stronger influx of 'Oxygen' especially for the 'Brain', which could result in bringing in some good benefits!

Our second option: <u>'Swing Low'</u>: could be for us, who like to be a bit more on the save-side; while exercising! We may simply swing into the 'Back-Rest-Position'; and with a bit good breathing and speaking some lovely Psalm-verses. Both options may turn out quite productive and enjoyable.

Some swings can bring us into our
Second Re-Run-with-Sit 'n' Push-next

EPISODE: 6 - Action!

"He only is my rock and my salvation; he is my defence;
I shall not be greatly moved." Psalm 62, 2

"Psalm: 126"!

When the LORD turned again the captivity of Zion, we were like them that dream.

Then was our mouth filled with laughter, and our tongue with singing: then said they among the heathen, The LORD has done great things for them.

The LORD has done great things for us; thereof we are glad.

Turn again our captivity, O LORD, as the streams in the south.

They that sow in tears shall reap in joy.

He that goes forth and weepeth, bearing precious seed, shall doubtless come again with rejoicing, bringing his sheaves with him.

Swing up into 'High' and hold position as long it is comfortable

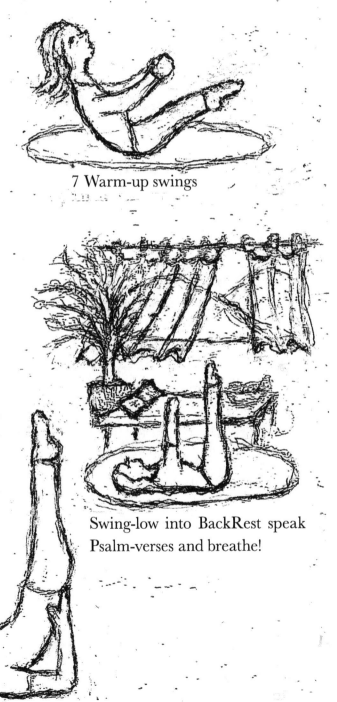

7 Warm-up swings

Swing-low into BackRest speak Psalm-verses and breathe!

Second-Re-Run and 'Sit 'n' Push'!

Presenting: <u>A Power-Combination</u>

Four basic 'Exercise-Positions' are working from one into the other, thereby creating a powerful-'work-out-combination'!

1) <u>The 'Pouch'</u> is rather interesting, because it can work simultaneous on some tummy muscles and back-muscles-all the way up to the neck and chin-area. It could be helpful to prevent in time – 'Double-Chin and Sagging' Effects'.
2) <u>The "Tummy Squeeze"</u> is always working hard to keep the mid-section strong and flat.
3) <u>The "Lower-Back-Lift"</u> is just so effective with 'Breathing' - It can greatly strengthen the Lower-Back-Muscles!
4) <u>The "Sit 'n' Push"</u> It can help-in time-to keep some 'Arm-and-Shoulder-Muscles' in good working-condition:

Re-Run II

"Thou hast commanded us to keep thy precepts diligently."
Psalm 119, 4

A Combination of Three!

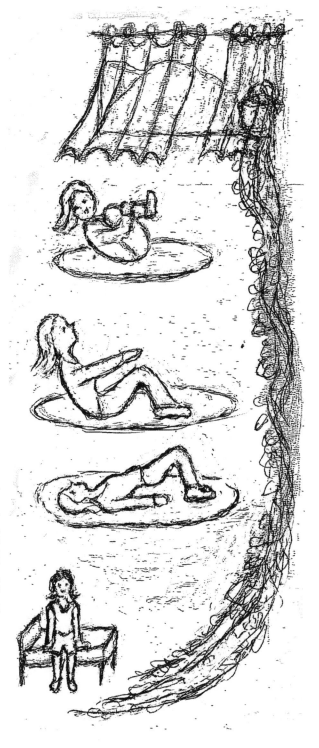

The Pouch: Cuddle up - breathe in deeply, hold breath-pouching cheeks- while lifting head and shoulders - while up, turn head to the right and blow a bit of air from the right corner of the mouth, turn head to the left and do the same in that direction, lay back down and breathe out completely.
(Repeat 7 times!)

The Tummy-squeeze: Lay back with knees pushed-up and feet placed on flat surface - with arms tended towards the knees push upper-torso quickly back and forth -:
(From 7 to 21 squeezes can have great results.)

The Lower-back-lift: Lay back with knees pushed-up and feet placed flat on surface: breathe in deeply while lifting your lower − back upwardly, hold position and breath while counting to seven: gently lower back down again while breathing out completely!
(Repeat procedure 7 times!)

The Sit 'n' Push: 20 to 30 Push-Ups can be sufficient

SCRIPT FOR EPISODE: 7

Presenting: <u>A Marvelous-Stretch!</u>

Wow! We are back on our feet now for the rest of our Episodes: Starting-out with a good stretch. Stretching is always good for the spine, and according to some Expert-Studies, Stretching can also strengthen the muscles on both sides of the chest, which are important to keep things on 'the up and up' and 'firm' in that area. All of which might be of 'Special-Interest' to some of our women-participants.

The Episode is winding down with 'Scoop-'n'-Loops'!

Let's just scoop down as far as we can! In time we will get better to do our loops and we'll yet enjoy a great exercise!

A few loops will bring us into our next Episode: 8

EPISODE: 7 - Action!

"Thus will I bless thee while I live, I will lift up my hands in thy name."
Psalm 63, 4

<u>A Marvelous Stretch with
Psalm 103:1-4</u>

Bless the LORD O my souls and all that is within me, bless his holy name.

Bless the LORD, O my soul, and forget not all his benefits.

Who forgiveth all thine inequities; who healeth all thy diseases.

Who Who redeemeth thy life from destruction; who crowneth thee with lovingkindness and tender mercies;

Stretch 'n' Breath and Speak Something 'Marvellous'!
Breathe-out completely after each stretch! (Repeat 4 to 5 times)

Follow-up with Scoop 'n' Loops!
Lean down-put in tummy - and touch the floor with our finger-then first-then with our mat bend to this expressly, tigh-hand-hips-head
(Repeat 4 to 5 times)

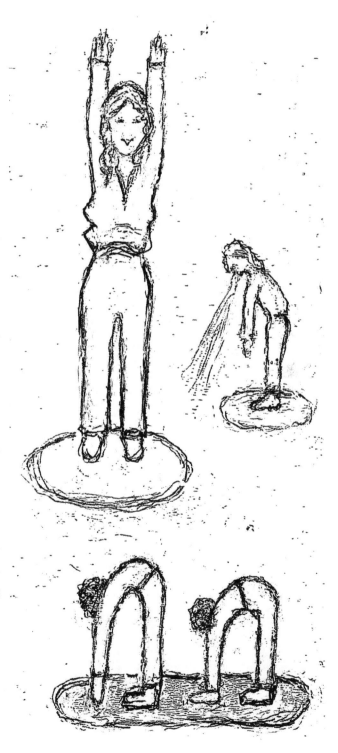

SCRIPT FOR EPISODE: 8

Presenting: <u>'Rock-'a' by Baby'</u>!

Wow! This 'Exercise' might go all the way back to "Mother Eve" Who had to work hard, while rocking two Babies back to sleep! Maybe 'Cain' didn't get enough rocking that's why he turned out such a 'Meany'! Ha!-just kidding!

'Attention' to all 'Moms and Dads' who are currently rocking their real 'Bundle of Joy'; they are hereby exempt from this exercise'! For they have done their good work already! This is according to some 'Expert'-studies; which maintain that 'Rocking' and 'Cuddling' are quite important - factors for Good-Child-Development'I Never fear!

'There is always the 'Blessing'!'

A few turns will bring us into our next Episode: 9

EPISODE 8 - Action!

"And now, LORD, what wait I for? my hope is in thee."
Psalm 39, 7

<u>Rock a by Baby!</u>

<u>Little things to remember that can bring the great results:</u>

1) Use any of the substitutes in place of Baby!
2) Hold object on a fairly high level with elbows spread outwardly.
3) Keep legs and feet somewhat apart,
4) Try to pull tummy in while swinging the object from side to side.

Between 20 and 40 swings, depending on progress, should bring some good results in the waist-line.

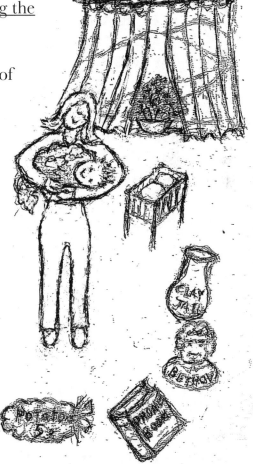

Substitute items can be used in place of Baby between 3 to 5 pound items can be sufficient!

SCRIPT FOR EPISODE: 9

Presenting: 'Ballet-Lessons'!

With Baby safely taken care of; Let's have some time-out to visit our friends at the 'Ballet-Studio', to join them for some 'Leg-exercising' with the uttermost charm of the 'Star-Ballerina'!

In case some of our male-participants would rather do their leg-stretching in a 'Sturdy Gym', that is quite alright!

In any case: With 'charm' or 'sturdiness', the exercise can be good for strengthening some leg-muscles from the toes up to the hips which could give us a new swing in our walk-making-way-for happy times to come!

A few kicks will get us right into Episode: 10

EPISODE: 9 - Action!

"Let them praise his name in the dance."
Psalm 149, 3

<u>Ballet-Lessons</u>

<u>Front – Kicks!</u>

Kick leg up with leg and foot stretched straight forward, pull tummy-in while kicking up, this will create more thrust and work for a stronger posture. Between 7 and 21 kicks can be sufficient for each leg.

<u>Back – Kicks!</u>

Kick leg back with your foot pulled into an-up-ward position; (the toe crunched up!)

Count again:
From 7 to 21 kicks
for each leg.

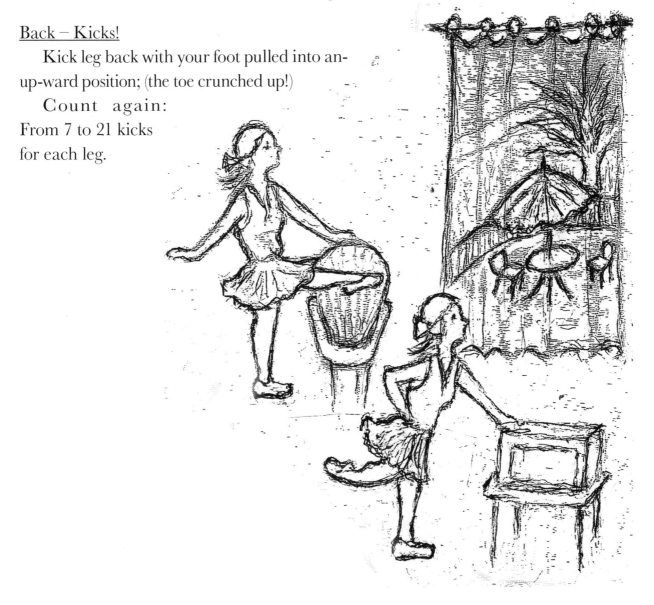

SCRIPT for EPISODE: 10

Presenting: <u>'Back-Home at the Ranch'</u>!

Wow! We can already see it from far! There is some work to do! Side-ways and walk-ways are full of glutter at the Ranch!

While doing a great cleaning-job, let's also get rid of some 'mental-glutter'!

Worries-angers-envies-rage-and other negatives; let's sweep them all out! Who needs them? They are nothing but the 'enemy'!

"The Little Foxes that spoil the wine"!

But let's also remember: When all is clean and empty; let's quickly fill-up again with lots of 'praising-praying'-and all kind of positive-stuff!

That will make it harder for the 'enemy' to come back-in again!

A few sweeps will bring us directly into Episode: 11

EPISODE 10 - Action!

"Then did I beat them small as the dust before the wind: I did cast them out as the dirt in the street." Psalm 18, 42

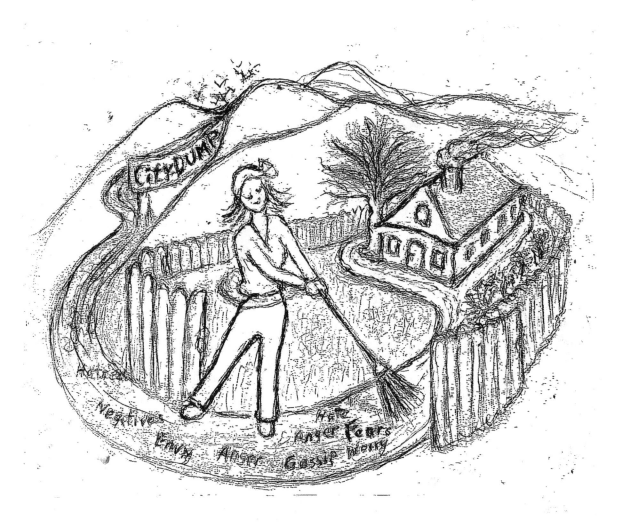

<u>Sweep - Out - Time!</u>

Let's clean-sweep our garden as well as our mind! Sweeping-out the negative clutter!

SCRIPT: Episode: 11

Presenting: <u>"Stretch and Speak"</u>!

    After all that work, Episode: 11 will quickly come to our aid again and feature for us another good - 'Stretching-Exercise'!

    The structure and technique will be the same as the exercise in Episode: 7; however a new selection of some delightful Psalm-verses will make the difference to create for us again another productive and enjoyable 'Exercising-Experience'!

    The 'Scoop 'n' Loops' will bring us directly into Episode: 12

Episode: 11 - Action!

"Mine eyes are eyes toward the LORD; for he shall pluck my feet out of the wet."
Psalm 25:15

<u>Stretch and Speak and Breath</u>
<u>Psalm 34 1-4</u>

I will bless the LORD at all times: his praise shall continually be in my mouth.

My soul shall make her boast in the LORD, the humble shall hear thereof, and be glad.

O magnify the LORD with me, and let us exalt his name together.

I souht the LORD, and he heard me, and delivered me from all my fears.

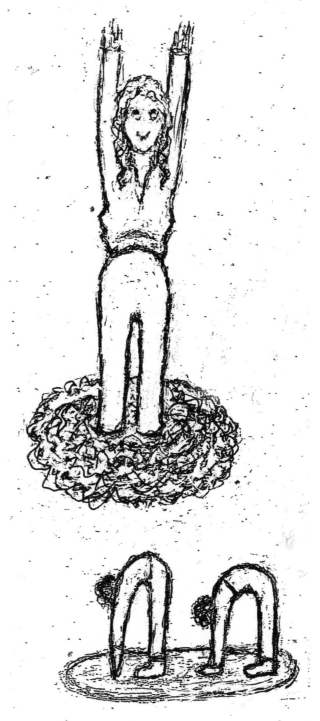

lets wind up with
scoops 'n' loops
Repeat 'stretch' about 4 times! while speaking some psalm-verses.

Follow-up with Scoop 'n' Loops
Stretch and breathe and speak some of the mindful Psalm verses. Look for guidelines in the headings-script of
Episode 7!

SCRIPT for EPISODE: 12

Presenting: <u>The Victory-Run!</u>

The Victory-Run was greatly inspired by a young American-Athlete: Who in her youth suffered a touch of 'paralysis' in her legs'. All her family started to pray; and she got better! In fact, she got so much better that she was now a member of a 'Running-Team' where she would make the most powerful-Training-Runs! Reporters were simply amazed! They were always asking her and wondering how she could do so great?

Finally on TV, in the midst of several reporters, the 'Little Girl' told them a bit about her life; about her trials and troubles and about her Wondres-Healing! And toward the end she said: "Now I just run for Jesus."

It is not so clear, how the reporters reacted at that time; maybe some rolled their eyes? But one thing is very clear: Our "Little Girl Wilma Rudolph" won her first 'Gold-Medal' of the-1960-'Olympic games' in ROME-ITALY! And she became one of the 'Great-Winners' in Olympic-History!

And so can we be; "Winners" - Not giving up but keep on walking or running for that great victory in time ahead!

"O sing unto the LORD a new song; for he hath done marvelous things."
Psalm: 98, 1

EPISODE 12 - Action!

"His right hand, and his holy arm hath gotten him the victory." Psalm 98, 1.

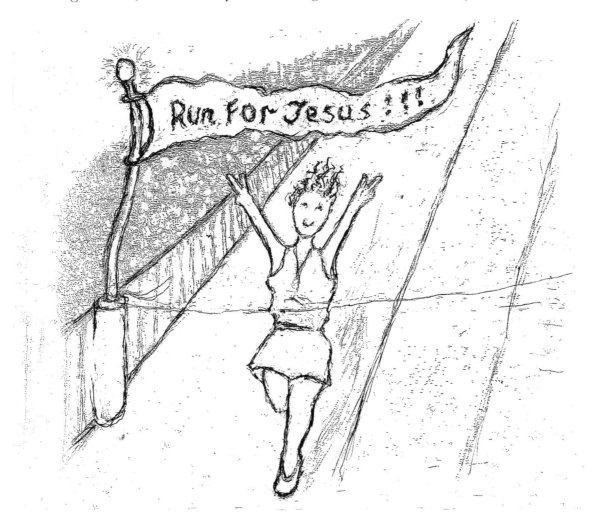

Stationary-Leaping or Walking!

Leaping happily or walking softly with 'Grace'. Whatever it's best for us! Counting to 20 with each finger of three-hands-full! (300-counts) With our last count of 20- let's make the Victory sign!

Little Gems for Health
"…and bread which strengtheneth man's heart."
Psalm: 104-15

Now, after our good work-out we may feel well and refreshed; so let's not forget a few good things to keep us going into the right direction!

1) Wow! Remember the 'Water'! Let's try to drink at least 3 to 4 small bottles of water-besides-tea, coffee and orange juice all this in one day!

2) Let's be smart and think before we eat! It might even be fun to find new and more valuable food to enjoy! Great magazines like "Woman's-world" has lots of wonderful information about 'Foods and Diets'!

3) Let's not forget our 'Daily-Bread'! Bread can give us great needed 'Fiber and according to modern studies: It is the 'Crust' of the bread that contains most of the B-Vitamins which are important for sustaining certain 'Brain-functions'! Bread has actually a long 'History' which may go back all the way, to 'Ancient-Nomadic-Tribes, who accidentally (or divinely) discovered certain 'wheat-patches' with fully-packed 'Special-Seeds'-ready for the wonder of 'Sowing and Reaping'! Wow! For all of us, and especially for the 'growing-young', it may be of great benefit to eat at least some 'Crusts' of that wonderful-stuff called "Bread" every day!

Little Gems for 'Beauty'
"…and oil to make his face to shine."
Psalm: 104-15

Wow! There is a 'Gem' on our tree already; our humble little 'Lime'! It is the juice of the 'Lime' with all that vitamin 'C' which can directly soak into the skin that is so great! Then, adding some drops of vitamin-E-OIL - and applying all this to our face, and perhaps a bit into our hair and 'Bresto'! We might come out beautiful! Shining like the Sun!

Another 'Little Gem': Our lushes California 'Avocado' has a Little 'Beauty-Secret' hidden right under its skin'! It is the oil which has been found quite nourishing! It may even prevent early wrinkling!

So now, we can happily eat our 'Toast and Avocado' first and save the 'skin' for later, to give ourselves a nice little 'facial'! We might look a bit 'green' for a while; so let's not forget to wash before going out!

There are surely many more Beauty-Gems to be found. But there is one 'Special-Beauty' that comes to us only from above, from our wonderful "Heavenly-Father" who loves us all so much!

"…he will beautify the meek with salvation."
Psalm: 149, 4.

Printed in the United States
By Bookmasters